Jason Roach, Philippa Taylor

FACING INFERTILITY

Guidance for Christian couples considering IVF

CMF
Christian Medical Fellowship

Facing Infertility
Guidance for Christian couples considering IVF

Published by Christian Medical Fellowship. 6 Marshalsea Road, London SE1 1HL
www.cmf.org.uk

ISBN 978-0-906747-51-3

ACKNOWLEDGEMENTS

From Jason:
To all those over the years that I have had the opportunity to counsel. Thank you for your honesty, your critiques and above all for teaching me more of what it looks like to trust God through adversity. I praise God for his work in you. May the comfort that he has given you be a blessing to others as you comfort them (2 Corinthians 1:3-4)

From Philippa:
If ever an issue needs both grace and truth this must be high up the list. As a part of the Christian Medical Fellowship team I have the privilege of being able to draw on both the professional expertise and knowledge, as well as the practical, caring experience of many members and friends of CMF, who have provided much needed input to our many drafts. We have been so grateful for this help and I hope that the result indeed reflects God's truth and love in equal measure.

ABOUT THE AUTHORS

Jason Roach worked as a medical doctor in Paediatrics and Intensive Care in London where he gained his Masters in Bioethics. He also worked for several years in academic medical journalism with the British Medical Journal. He is currently a full time Anglican minister working in Westminster and with London City Mission on a housing estate in Battersea.

Philippa Taylor is Head of Public Policy at the Christian Medical Fellowship and is a Consultant on Family and Bioethics to Christian Action Research and Education (CARE). She has an Masters in Bioethics from St Mary's University and for the past twenty or so years has been speaking, writing and working in public policy on a wide range of contemporary bioethical issues.

The views expressed in this booklet are solely those of the authors and do not claim to represent those of Christian Medical Fellowship, or any of the academic institutions or other organisations with which the authors are affiliated.

Christian Medical Fellowship

Christian Medical Fellowship is a network of doctors and medical students in the UK, connected to over 80 national Christian medical organisations around the world. Many CMF members are involved in International Health, and some are working long-term in less developed countries.

CONTENTS

1. INTRODUCTION

Infertility affects about one in seven couples and is often deeply distressing, affecting every area of life. The options available are complex and confusing. On the one hand couples are faced with the reality that relatively few babies are available for adoption. On the other hand there are now myriad ways in which they can have their own, or even someone else's, child.

In light of this it can be difficult for married Christian couples to think through the ethics of in vitro fertilisation (IVF), an option most will consider when struggling with infertility.[1] This guidance is designed to provide some help for individuals considering IVF and for churches wanting to offer support for such couples.

There are many more personal scenarios and technological options than can be fully discussed in a short booklet. Therefore we do not consider this guidance a replacement for individual discussion with both church leaders and doctors.

IVF encompasses several different techniques. Most of this guidance, however, deals with the basic IVF technique. This involves fertilising eggs and sperm outside of the womb in order to implant embryos back into the womb. We do not discuss in detail the biological background to infertility, although there is a glossary of terms and pointers to further resources at the end. The issues involved mean that in places there are complex ethical questions to address. This is unavoidable given what is at stake. We therefore apologise in advance if the tone of this guidance seems insensitive at any point. It is merely our attempt to explain the issues as clearly as possible. With this in mind, we have included two personal testimonies from couples who both considered IVF and decided to take different courses of action for themselves.[2]

2. A DESIRE FOR CHILDREN

The desire to have children of our own is natural, legitimate and good. Several Bible passages recognise the pain and loneliness of infertility.[3] However, like any desire, we must guard against it becoming unhealthily strong. A desire to have a child 'at any cost' is neither spiritually or emotionally healthy.[4] It is important to remember that a marriage in which there are no children is in no way invalid or 'second class.' Although children are a blessing rightly anticipated within marriage, they are not essential to it and a marriage is complete without them.

One option that couples are not often aware of is Natural Procreative Technology (NaProTechnology). NaProTechnology tries as far as possible to diagnose underlying causes and manage the various factors that can make infertility more likely. It is far less invasive than IVF and not ethically problematic.[5] Two recent studies have shown that NaProTechnology produced successful pregnancy in comparable proportions to IVF and further research is on-going.[6]

We would strongly encourage couples to consider adoption alongside deliberations about IVF. It is possible to have a healthy, loving family without any genetic link between parents and child. Adoption is a wonderful act of rescue mirroring God's loving adoption of us.[7] We recognise that the process of adopting a baby carries its own emotional challenges. However, as well as providing a loving home for a child who is in need, adoption avoids the ethical complications of assisted reproductive technology. We also acknowledge that in reality few babies are available for adoption nowadays, so adoption of older children or children with special needs is likely to be a more realistic option, and this can be a highly challenging, if ultimately rewarding, option for couples. There is a personal testimony in the appendix from one couple who pursued the option of adoption.

A diversity of opinion in medical and theological perspectives means that these guidelines are written with a humble attitude on what is a complex issue. Nevertheless, despite some inevitable disagreement, we are committed to the fact that the Bible equips us for all we need to live godly lives, and it supplies us with the ethical principles necessary to discern the wisest course of action.[8] These biblical principles should provide the starting point and grounding for any thinking about infertility treatments for Christians.

3. WHAT DOES THE BIBLE SAY ABOUT INFERTILITY AND IVF?

Applying the Bible to contemporary medical problems is always challenging because we cannot simply look up words like 'IVF' and 'embryo' in a concordance. Nonetheless there are clear biblical principles that can help us negotiate the minefield and find an approach that is consistent with both God's compassion and his commands.

First, we must remember that God has a deep concern for those who face infertility and the heartbreak that it brings. Abraham and Sarah had to wait longer than they felt able before their promised son, Isaac, was born.[9] Similarily Hannah's anguished prayer, weeping and refusal to eat illustrates the stress of infertility.[10] The inclusion of these stories shows that God is aware of the pain that an unfulfilled desire for children may cause.

However God is not just concerned – he is sovereignly in control.[11] The Scriptures tell us that all human beings belong to him.[12] He then graciously entrusts children to us as gifts.[13] We may yearn for change in our situation but none of us has a right to demand such a gift. Infertility and fertility are not the results of random chance events determined by an accidental roll of the dice. It is the all-knowing and loving God, who even sent his Son to die for us, who is in control of both.

God's 'creation mandate' is for humans to 'fill the earth and subdue it.'[14] This stewardship process is not a licence to exploit the world but a commission to use it in service to God. Many Christians understand scientific enquiry and its application as part of this. In other words, God has given us the ability to discover and apply all kinds of technological innovations in creative new ways for the purpose of helping other human beings. Healthcare is one way in which we can help to repair some of the physical effects of living in a fallen world. Most Christians thereby regard medicine, used correctly, as a God-given gift. Accordingly, we can and should use our God-given skills to help alleviate infertility.[15]

However, just because we have developed a particular technology does not mean that it is necessarily right to use it. When a discovery or invention violates a biblical moral principle it will be wrong to use it.

The biblical account of creation treats marriage, sexual intercourse and reproduction as ordinarily linked together. The Bible is clear that these are rightly to be considered within marriage. As we work through the specific issues raised by IVF we will explore them within this biblical context. There will be some couples who, for reasons of personal conscience, will choose a more cautious path than the one we believe that the Bible permits. We encourage church members to support couples emotionally and practically if that is the case for them.

4. WHEN IS IVF CONSIDERED?

Couples considering IVF are normally advised that before approaching their GP about getting help with infertility, they should have been trying for a baby by having regular unprotected sex for two years.[16] At this stage, a medical check is done to get as much information as possible. This may include physical examinations, tests to check blood hormone levels, ovarian function and sperm quality and scans of the reproductive organs. Sometimes keyhole surgery or an X-ray with special dye is performed to pick up anything that a normal scan may miss, such as blockages or adhesions (internal organs sticking together) in the pelvic cavity.

Consideration of lifestyle factors is also necessary, as these can be important in optimising the chances of treatment success (for example, smoking and alcohol consumption). Taking folic acid (vitamin) supplements is usually advised.

Although there are recommended levels of funding for IVF treatment, actual funding and the criteria for accessing it will vary by region.[17]

What does IVF involve?

The main IVF technique involves giving the woman fertility drugs to stimulate egg production, and then surgically retrieving the eggs from the ovaries by keyhole surgery or using an ultrasound guide.[18] She is then given hormones to prepare her womb for pregnancy, while the eggs are fertilised with the sperm in a laboratory. A maximum of two embryos are then implanted into the woman's womb and, if all goes well, a normal pregnancy is achieved.[19]

Intracytoplasmic Sperm Injection (ICSI) is now used almost as often as IVF for infertility treatment.[20] ICSI follows the same procedure as above, but the sperm is directly injected to the egg, rather than being left to its own devices. ICSI is used especially for men for whom the standard IVF technique would fail, for example if their sperm are unable to penetrate the egg or there are other significant abnormalities with the sperm.

How successful is IVF?

One of the main factors influencing the outcome of IVF treatment is the age of the woman whose eggs are used, as the quality of the eggs declines as the woman gets older. In 2010 the percentage of IVF cycles started that resulted in a live birth was 32% for women aged under 35 years, dropping to 5% for women aged between 43-44 years and 1.9% for women aged 45 and over.[21] The women who have the best chance of becoming pregnant are usually those aged 37 and under, who are on their first or second attempt at IVF. The rate of birth defects, chromosome abnormality or miscarriage also rises with maternal age.[22]

5. WHAT PRACTICAL AND ETHICAL ISSUES ARE RAISED?

1. Risks to mothers

There is limited evidence that IVF involves a certain amount of risk to the mother.[23] However, it is important to view the risks realistically. *Any* medical treatment involves risk. The question that always needs to be asked is *how does that risk compare with doing nothing?* Clearly, for example, risks equivalent to natural childbirth would be acceptable if IVF is otherwise acceptable. Over and above this, different couples may come to different conclusions based on their circumstances just as they might for other, less controversial, medical procedures. For example, a very risky operation to repair the hand of a concert pianist may seem more acceptable in his/her case than it would for others. Someone with cancer will be more willing to accept the burdens of chemotherapy in view of the potential benefits. We realise that the emotional and relational consequences of infertility are significant and personal to every couple.

'*The single greatest health risk for women conceiving following fertility treatment is a multiple pregnancy*'.[24] The risk of early and late miscarriage is higher with a multiple pregnancy, as is the risk of high blood pressure. During birth, mothers of twins are more likely to require extra medical care.[25] In addition, an ectopic pregnancy can still occur after IVF. This is when an embryo develops in a woman's fallopian tube rather than her womb. Ectopic pregnancy can cause vaginal bleeding and low pregnancy hormone levels and leads to miscarriage. It can also lead in very rare cases to bleeding which can be life-threatening.

The risk of multiple births is reduced by transferring fewer embryos. The most common number of embryos transferred in each treatment cycle is two; (60% of women received a double embryo transfer in 2011). 36% of women received a single embryo transfer, although half of these took place because only one embryo was available to transfer.[26]

Other risks to the mother come from the use of high doses of drugs to stimulate the ovaries for egg production. This can generate mild reactions, such as hot flushes, feeling down or irritable, headaches and restlessness.[27] However the drugs can also cause ovarian hyper-stimulation syndrome (OHSS), with symptoms such as chest pains, shortness of breath and, occasionally leads to kidney failure and death.[28] Approximately one in 100 to one in 200 patients will need a stay in hospital because of OHSS.

2. Risks to babies

The process itself

There is evidence to suggest that the rate of birth defects may be slightly higher for babies born via ICSI and IVF.[29] However the Human Fertilisation and Embryology Authority (HFEA) states that this risk is low.[30]

As with mothers, there are also risks to children born from a multiple pregnancy: '*It increases the risk of stillbirth, neonatal death and disability in children born.*'[31] At least half of all twins are born several weeks earlier than singleton babies and so they weigh less and are more likely to experience serious health problems. Twins are also up to six times more likely to die within the first 28 days of life than singletons.[32] Again, the numbers actually affected are still small.

We view the risk of injury to the embryo differently to that of risk to the mother since the child involved is exposed to it *without their consent*. However, it is important to be aware that in the case of a fertile couple having sex approximately 50% of embryos die naturally before a woman is even aware that she is pregnant.[33] Sex is an expected norm of marriage despite this reality (eg 1 Corinthians 7:5). Given this, the uncomfortable reality is that, in a fallen world, embryo loss in the course of normal sexual intercourse is considered by God to be acceptable.[34] It is impossible to ascertain precisely the rate of either natural loss or loss in IVF and both will vary between individuals and fertility clinics. However, we would suggest that the risk of artificially implanting created embryos into the womb involves a risk which is of a similar order to that which occurs naturally, making it acceptable *in principle.*[35] This is simply replicating the normal contingencies under God's sovereignty inside the womb.[36]

Some have argued that IVF is fundamentally unnatural and leads to treating children as *means* rather than *ends* in themselves. In other words, considering children valuable merely for how they can benefit us, rather than valuable in their own right. Although this is possible, we have already made the point that using healthcare creatively to repair the physical effects of the fall is legitimate. It is, in our view, simply an application of God's command at creation to 'subdue' and 'rule' over the earth. It is difficult to argue conclusively that the numbers involved automatically lead to a general change in attitude over procreation.

This means that IVF, as a process, is in principle ethically acceptable.[37]

Spare embryos

IVF usually generates spare embryos as normally more eggs are fertilised per treatment than are implanted as embryos. This is not, however, a compulsory or necessary component of IVF, although clearly producing spare embryos may increase the chances of a successful pregnancy and hence reduce the costs involved.[38]

The production of spare embryos raises one of the most important decisions Christians need to make about IVF. Spare embryos that are not implanted into the womb are instead 1) used for research, 2) discarded, or 3) frozen for future use. Freezing compromises embryo survival and there is a high possibility that frozen embryos will never be used by the parents.

Our society thinks that because human embryos are (at best) small, weak and physically insignificant they are expendable. But this conflicts with how most Christians understand the biblical principles on early human life.

The developing life in the womb may be small, but each embryo is fully human, made in the image of God and therefore deserves the utmost respect, care and protection (Genesis 1:26-27, 9:6; James 3:9). This is not only a responsibility required by the sixth commandment but part of our mandate to champion care for the weak and the vulnerable (Psalm 82:3-4, Isaiah 1:17).

The issue of when human life first begins has been the subject of much debate. The Bible, however, is clear that God is involved in human life before birth. Other than controversial interpretations of Exodus 21:22-25 [39] there is nothing else in Scripture that even remotely suggests that the unborn child or embryo is anything other than a human person from the time of conception. According to Luke 1:30-35, the life story of Jesus Christ on earth began when he was conceived by Mary, through the Holy Spirit. Matthew records that the angel tells Joseph: '*...what is conceived in her is from the Holy Spirit.*' (Matthew 1:20). God became incarnate as an embryo. The implications of this are profound. There can be no doubt that Jesus' human life – his personal identity – began at the point of conception, in the womb of Mary. The identification of his 'becoming flesh' with his mother's act of conception thus demonstrates both the humanity and personal nature of the early embryo. [40]

Although it is impossible to say categorically whether this extends back to the moment of fertilisation, the burden of proof is on those who want to disprove this assumption. If one was out hunting deer and saw what could be a deer or a human and decided to shoot, that person would be responsible for their actions should it turn out to be a human! The fact that the Old Testament legislated against accidental killing means that we should seek to avoid even the risk of harm (Numbers 35:22-28; Deuteronomy 19:4ff).

In the light of the biblical testimony on life before birth we believe that we should give the embryo the benefit of any doubt that we think still exists (Ecclesiastes 11:5). Unless we can be *sure* that the embryo is not fully human, then we should show it the utmost respect (Romans 14:23), whatever the personal cost may be. [41]

We therefore advise against the intentional creation of spare embryos since at the present time their creation involves the inevitable destruction of some. Although we have stated that many embryos are lost 'naturally' when fertile couples have sex, this fact cannot be used to condone *deliberately destroying spare embryos*. This is because nature cannot be used as a universal moral benchmark. Many people die in natural disasters such as floods, earthquakes and famine. This does not mean these people are any less valuable or worthy of protection. These natural tragedies cannot reliably guide us as to how we treat *individuals in other situations*. What happens naturally inside the womb cannot govern how we ought to treat embryos *intentionally* outside of the womb.[42]

The implications for IVF are that it is ethically problematic to allow spare embryos to be destroyed or used for research.

Freezing and thawing embryos also exposes them to unnecessary extra risk. This becomes an issue when more embryos are produced than can be implanted into the womb at one time (UK guidance stipulates a maximum of two in most circumstances).[43] An NHS clinical knowledge summary suggests that: '*not all embryos will survive freezing and eventual thawing when they come to be used. Very occasionally no embryos will survive.*'[44] Studies vary in what they perceive the success rate to be but the majority cite a two-thirds success rate for the freeze-thaw process. Given the current failure rate, freezing embryos seems to us the equivalent to taking three children to another country knowing that one will not survive the journey. It is difficult to conceive of many scenarios in which undertaking this level of risk voluntarily would be acceptable.[45] We note that the risk involved is changing as research continues.

In our view, at the present time, freeze-thawing exposes embryos to unnecessary extra risk and so is ethically problematic.[46]

If embryos are inadvertently created, the most ethical way forward would seem to be to make every effort to transfer them to the mother. This is because leaving them frozen indefinitely would be ethically unacceptable and the long term risks of freezing are unknown. Recent developments in egg freezing may thankfully make the need for embryo freezing increasingly rare.[47]

6. WIDER ETHICAL ISSUES

Masturbation[48]

The Bible does not address masturbation directly but does deal extensively with the issue of lust and the intended nature of sex. Lust is the 'desire to engage in sexual acts that are contrary to God's law (ie not in the context of a loving relationship between husband and wife).'[49] This is expressly forbidden by Jesus (Matthew 5:25-27 cf Genesis 3:6). However the IVF context does not *necessarily* fall under Jesus' prohibition. In this case masturbation could be focused entirely on the sexual attractiveness of your wife with her full awareness and even involvement. In this situation masturbation is in no way a secret and selfish act that ignores the fact that sex is intended to be relational. For those uncomfortable with this conclusion, however, there are also special semen collection condoms available that avoid the issue altogether.

Donated gametes

In the Bible, Genesis 2:24 sets out the basic framework of marriage: a lifelong commitment between a man and a woman that is based on leaving, cleaving and becoming 'one flesh'.[50] In Matthew 19:4-6 and Mark 10:6-9, Jesus confirms that marriage is part of the created order. The Bible clearly teaches that marriage is the only proper context for sexual intercourse and also God's ideal for raising children.[51] So does the use of donor eggs or sperm somehow violate this marriage relationship?

In some ways using donated eggs or sperm does introduce another person into the marital relationship. Since the intrusion is primarily genetic and not social (the donor is normally anonymous) it may not be right to call this adultery as some have done.[52] Moreover, using donor gametes does not involve intercourse outside the marriage relationship nor the cheating and lust aspects of an adulterous relationship. However, it does disturb the exclusive nature of the marriage bond (Genesis 2:24, Matthew 19:5-6).[53] John Stott described it as an '*intrusion into the bonds of marriage and parenthood.'*[54] Donor gametes, whether egg or sperm, introduce a third person who will be genetically related to the child, but will play no part in their upbringing. Effectively removing one partner from the genetic equation may also breed resentment or jealousy in the relationship with partner and child. In addition, the effects on the child in terms of difficulties with identity are becoming better known as more children speak out about being deprived of their genetic link and knowledge of their biological heritage and identity.[55]

Therefore, we have deep reservations about the use of donated gametes and strongly advise against their use for infertility treatment.

Donated embryos

It is important to be aware that donation of an embryo in effect relinquishes control over their destiny. However, *accepting* a donated embryo is essentially a very early adoption. It is a means of caring for some of the weakest members of our society and may also avoid them being subject to destructive research or indefinite storage.

Surrogacy

Superficially, surrogacy may appear to be a possible response to the pain of a childless couple. However, surrogacy takes no regard for the basic presumption that a child's best interest is to be born into a natural family structure in which the family relationships have not been intentionally confused. The child and the surrogate, the most vulnerable parties and the most likely to be harmfully affected, receive little or no protection.

There are two cases of surrogacy in the Bible, both of which illustrate the distortion of family relationships and society that can result. (Abram and Sarah, using Hagar, and Rachel and Jacob, using Bilhah[56]). This should give us reason for caution since the outcomes were jealousy, rivalry, favouritism and discord within the family. However there are certain medical scenarios in which a woman may not be able to physically carry a child to term and another woman is sacrificially willing to do so. While this introduces a third party it does not do so in such a way as to significantly impact the genetic parenthood of the child (though it will have a social effect). Couples should be aware that this option is fraught with difficulty for practical and ethical reasons, for the surrogate as well as the child and couple. Pursuing surrogacy may be possible but we believe it is unwise and adoption would be a far more preferable option. The legalities of surrogacy arrangements in the UK, as well as some of the practical and ethical concerns with it are dealt with in greater detail in the *CMF File*, 'Surrogacy'.[57]

In our view, Christians should be prepared to say no to surrogacy arrangements.

Research

We lament the fact that research takes place on human embryos, one of the most vulnerable points of human life. We would rather that this stopped now *even if* it would improve the effectiveness of infertility treatment. However this does not necessarily mean that Christians cannot and should not benefit from research that has been done already (for example, in having their already-created IVF embryos implanted). The Bible gives many examples of God's people benefitting from pagan knowledge when used for the service of God.[58] As long as our actions do not *in themselves* or *as a direct consequence* harm embryos, we may be able do them without being associated with the sin of those who perform research on embryos. We would encourage Christian couples embarking on IVF to be open about their grave reservations about embryo research for the sake of clarifying for others who may be confused or misunderstand their actions.

Costs

On average, one cycle of IVF costs about £5,000 at a private fertility clinic. However, this varies from clinic to clinic and there are likely to be additional costs for medicines, consultations and tests. IVF carries a failure rate between 67-97%, depending on the age of the woman and the cause of the infertility.[59] Even with several cycles of treatment there is no guarantee of success. This will inevitably exhaust the resources of many of the couples who are unable to get NHS treatment. The significant costs need to be weighed carefully against other stewardship considerations. There is no right answer. Couples will have very different personal circumstances but it would be sensible to discuss the issue with trusted Christian friends. In addition the emotional rollercoaster of raised hopes and dashed expectations is another important cost to be considered.

Conscience

We have covered a substantial amount of ethical ground. It is quite possible that on any number of issues you feel uncomfortable about proceeding with IVF or other forms of assisted reproductive technology. We would urge you not to proceed with IVF or any other fertility treatment if you are conflicted in your conscience as to whether it is right or wrong. The Apostle Paul reminds us that to do what we *believe* to be wrong is indeed wrong for us regardless of what others might think (Romans 14:13-17).

7. CONCLUSIONS

- Be of one mind as to the course of action you decide to take. As hard as it might be, aim to discuss even the most intimate details of the procedure openly and honestly.

- Remember that God stands with us in the brokenness of our world, aware of our pain and asking us to respond in faith.

- Be aware that the ethical issues are often more complex in practice than in theory. You may be asked to make quick decisions that you feel uncomfortable with. Try and be as clear as possible on what is ethically acceptable so as not to be pressured into decisions you are unsure about. Don't be afraid to say that you need time to think things through.

- Do your utmost to avoid going against your conscience.

- It is wise to consider less ethically problematic alternatives such as Natural Procreative Technology *prior* to considering IVF. For some couples this provides a non-invasive and cheaper alternative to IVF.[60]

- It is wise to consider less ethically problematic (although by no means easier) alternatives such as adoption *while* considering IVF. Adoption is a biblical pattern which profoundly expresses the love and grace of God (Romans 8:14-15; Galatians 4:1-7; Ephesians 1:3-6).

- If a couple choose IVF it would be wise to:

    - Be clear on what you have given consent for the clinic to do with any embryos that are created with regards to storage, donation and research.

    - Make provision for the care of inadvertently produced unused embryos in the event of death or health problems preventing further cycles.

- Avoid the use of donor gametes or embryos.
- See if the clinic can offer egg freezing as an alternative to embryo freezing.[61]

■ During the process be clear that:

- You would like all viable created embryos to be implanted in that cycle.[62]
- You would not like embryos to be created for the purpose of freezing in the first instance.
- You would like all those involved in the process to be aware of the special concerns and priorities you have.

■ Know when to stop trying:

- It can be helpful to think about the stopping point before starting treatment. It is not necessarily a negative approach; it simply means taking a realistic look at success rates and how far you are prepared to go to get a baby.[63]

■ Help others know how to support you:

- Church members are often ill-equipped to care for couples with infertility. You can help by suggesting what is most appropriate for you. For example, rather than suffering in silence when people offer platitudes, you can let them know the encouragements, prayers and acts of kindness that have been most comforting.[64]

8. TESTIMONIES

Ben and Corinne's story

We discovered that we were infertile by accident. Corinne was having a scan following a period of illness. The scanner just happened to mention that it looked as though her fallopian tubes were blocked. We had begun trying to get pregnant just a few months earlier so it was something of a shock to learn that our efforts were almost certainly in vain.

We were referred to a consultant in the Reproductive Medicine Unit at University College Hospital, London. She was very gentle and sensitive to the pain we were feeling. She explained the series of tests that they could perform to assess our fertility and the timescale involved. Everything seemed very drawn out. It was over a year until the tests were completed. They confirmed Corinne's fallopian tubes were blocked making conception humanly impossible.

Corinne has always longed to be a mummy. She doesn't have big career aspirations and had said for years that what she would really like to do is 'bake cakes, make babies, and tell people about Jesus.' The 'making babies' bit was a key component of her dreams. So it was especially hard for her. What made it particularly hard was being part of a congregation that seemed to be going through a baby boom. We struggled to understand why God was withholding this blessing from us and felt quite isolated in our pain. Looking back it would have been so helpful to have had an older Christian couple to meet, talk, pray and weep with us. By God's grace, our struggles with childlessness never brought tension between us. Following the tests we were referred to the Assisted Conception Unit (ACU) at Guy's Hospital and invited to attend an open evening.

At that stage we weren't sure what we thought about IVF ethically. We just felt a general suspicion. However, we decided to attend the evening to find out more. There were about 100 people present. Some members of the unit explained the process involved in the different treatments. We were given a pile of paperwork explaining everything in more detail.

We made an appointment to see one of the doctors individually. Before the appointment we read through the paperwork and found some helpful articles on the CMF website. It was clear that a normal round of treatment involved producing about a dozen embryos, transferring the best two to the woman's womb, with the rest frozen for possible future use. We definitely didn't want to create surplus embryos. We couldn't be sure we would be able to use them and were convinced it would be wrong to intentionally put our children's lives at such risk. We struggled with the thought of engaging in a treatment that was so immoral in its normal form.

Whether or not we were directly involved in sinful activity, we struggled with the idea of being treated by doctors who were engaged in destroying human life. One of our church ministers helped us to realise that association with sinful people does not mean we share in their guilt. The decision of whether to go ahead with IVF treatment was not one we took lightly.

We searched the Scriptures and prayed hard. For a long time it would have been wrong for us to proceed acting against our conscience, but over a period of a few months we agreed it was a good and right course of action for us to take. The desire to have children is a good one. We couldn't see any reason why it would be wrong, in principle, to use both money and medical technology to pursue that desire.

We went to the meeting at the ACU keen to discover if it would be possible for us to undergo the treatment without the risk of embryos being discarded. The doctor we saw was very understanding – both of our struggles with childlessness and of our Christian convictions about the status of embryos. She talked through how they could accommodate our wishes. This would involve giving Corinne a lower dose of drugs to produce fewer eggs, then attempting to fertilise just two eggs and, if they fertilised, transferring both to Corinne's womb. She did point out that this would dramatically reduce our chances of conception. If we had a failed attempt we would have to pay the full amount again for any future rounds of treatment.

The doctor said she would raise our case at the next department meeting to confirm that they would be happy to proceed in the way she had outlined. It seemed as though we were the first people to ever request such an adjustment to the treatment. Throughout our treatment the hospital staff were brilliant. Only one doctor expressed her disagreement with our convictions - making it clear she thought we were crazy to reduce our chances of pregnancy to protect these embryos. 'They're not really human, you know!'

After the initial consultation we received a letter summarising our conversation and confirming the unit would be willing to proceed in the way we had discussed. The next issue was when we could start. At that time the NHS funded one cycle of IVF for infertile couples, but it could take up to 18 months to reach the top of the waiting list. If we paid for a cycle ourselves we could start immediately. Timing was a factor because Corinne had a complication with her one remaining ovary meaning there was a possibility it would need to be removed. We therefore decided to proceed with a privately funded cycle of treatment. The total cost, including the drugs, was about £2,000. As things worked out, just as the treatment began we were given the NHS funding and so had our fee reimbursed.

The cycle of treatment took about a month in total and involved seven or eight visits to the unit. There was an initial appointment and scan to check that Corinne was at the right stage in her period and to demonstrate how to administer the drugs - daily nasal sprays and injections. It helped that Corinne was working as a nurse, so the injections were not as traumatic as they might be for others. After nine days, regular trips to the unit assessed the growth of follicles on Corinne's ovary. Once they were nearing optimum size, the day of egg collection was set - usually about day 15. That morning I had to produce some sperm in a small pot. The unit have a special room with a box full of porn magazines. I decided I could do without them. The egg collection procedure involved Corinne being sedated and then a large needle and tube was used to collect the eggs from her ovary. It was a pretty uncomfortable experience for Corinne but the staff at the unit gave excellent care. Two eggs were chosen at random (it is impossible to judge quality at this stage) and put in a dish together with my sperm. After some time for Corinne to recover from the sedation, we travelled home and waited till the next day to hear if the eggs had fertilised.

It was an emotional 24 hours. We wondered what was happening back at the unit – longing and praying that God would be at work to create life and waiting nervously by the phone the following morning. To our delight we learnt both eggs had fertilised. We rejoiced that by God's grace and power we had two children living in a dish at Guy's hospital.

On the next day we returned for what they call 'embryo transfer'. It was much quicker and simpler than the egg collection. They basically squirted the embryos through a tube into Corinne's womb. Corinne's reaction was to want to lie upside down for two weeks, fearing that they might fall out. Apparently that can't happen. However, those two weeks were nerve-wracking as we waited to discover if the lives God had created would implant in Corinne's womb. This part of the treatment has the highest drop-off rate. It's easy to get caught up with the percentages. Of course, our Father does not work to percentages and so we prayed earnestly that he would preserve the life of our children. Corinne rested a lot during those weeks, only doing what was necessary.

Due to her medical condition, Corinne needed a blood test to see if she was pregnant. She had the test in the morning and we then drove to the West Country for the start of the summer camp we were helping to lead, expecting to get the results that afternoon. Sadly they weren't able to process the results that day. But the following morning Corinne had a major bleed. The phone call we then received confirmed that the embryos had not implanted. It was a desperately sad day. We had invested so much – time, money, and energy – and it had failed.

The whole process of going through IVF involved a big investment of time and emotional energy. It meant that we were pretty blinkered for the duration of the treatment. During our first cycle of treatment only half a dozen people in addition to our families knew what we were doing. When that ended in miscarriage we decided we wanted to be more open. So for the second cycle we had an email list of 30 or so people who we asked to pray for us right from the start.

We felt that infertility and miscarriage were such unspoken topics that we wanted to try and address that by speaking openly about our experiences. Sometimes the fact we were using IVF treatment met with surprise. We had to give a lengthy explanation of how we were adjusting the treatment to make it ethically acceptable. Our experience has meant we've been able to advise and encourage a number of other couples who are going through similar struggles.

To complete the story, we undertook another cycle of IVF nine months after Corinne's miscarriage. We began the treatment thinking that if it failed again it would be our last attempt. The emotional drain of going through a failed cycle was such that we couldn't face doing it again. There was also the significant financial cost of undergoing treatment. In addition we had begun thinking seriously about adoption as a possibility and, while we felt that it would require a different attitude to having children biologically, we saw it as a good and godly alternative for us.

The result of our second cycle was that once again both eggs fertilised. God created two girls, Moya and Elsie, on 18 February 2005. Miraculously they both implanted in Corinne's womb. They were born by emergency C-section at 32 weeks, but sadly Elsie died 30 hours later.

Moya is now four years old and has a little sister, Darcy, who was also conceived through a third cycle of IVF. For that final cycle we requested that the unit only fertilise one egg to avoid the risk of another twin pregnancy. God was very kind and Darcy was conceived and safely born. We have decided not to pursue any further IVF treatment despite our desire to have more children. However, we are keen to explore the possibility of adoption at a later date.

As to the children of the first miscarriage, at the time we weren't sure quite how to think about the lives God had made. They had lived so briefly, yet we believed them to be our children with full human dignity. We weren't sure what form our grief should take. It was several years later that we decided to name them James and Hetty. We don't know what sex they were but a boy and girl seemed appropriate and we wanted to do something to acknowledge them as people.

We do think about them differently to our daughter Elsie, who was born just over a year later, and who died 30 hours after being born; just as we would think differently about one of our surviving daughters were they to die now. I think that is inevitable. But we trust that we will see them in the new creation and find out if our gender guesses were right!

We thank God that the medical technology existed to enable us to become parents. Our experiences were tough at times but we can see how God has used them to shape us and hopefully make us useful to others.

Sam and Anne's story

As I write it is a windy autumn day, and our three-year-old twin daughters are full of excitement over conkers, acorns, the big storm last night, pretend tea parties, fairies, why you can't actually see Jesus like you can see Mummy and Daddy, how and why cheese melts and a thousand other things. We are in the process of picking schools for them, as they start Reception next September. All very normal! Yesterday we had a visit from the girls' big sister, who is six, and her parents, who we were meeting for the first time. Not so normal! Like our girls, their sister has been adopted but into a different family, for various reasons. With inquisitive little girls, the story of how we got to our current state of mostly normal with smatterings of extremely abnormal comes up naturally in daily life, but some aspects of it seem like they happened in the dim and distant past.

The year after we were married, my husband Sam had a testicle removed after weeks of extreme pain, labelled at times an infection and at others torsion. Although assured by doctors it would not affect our fertility, we began to consider the possibility that conceiving a child might not be as straightforward as we'd assumed. At the time we were in a prayer group with a couple who were struggling with infertility and being assessed for adoption, so even at that early stage this option was at the back of our minds. The doctors suggested getting a sperm test if we were concerned, but for a number of reasons we did not do this right away. In retrospect it's clear that God's timing was right in terms of when we started investigations.

We started to try for children in December 2007. After nothing had happened six months on, we went to the GP who said to wait a few more months. We were concerned my cycle might be irregular in some ways and went back to start the first round of tests later that year. A sperm test revealed that no sperm was present in the sample, and the doctor informed us that this meant we couldn't have children. The doctor asked us to redo the test, so we then had an agonising week waiting for the result to be either confirmed or overturned, praying hard both for the first test to have been wrong but also for God's help to trust him if it was right. Sadly, the result was confirmed, and we were referred to a fertility specialist to investigate further. That was December 2008, a rather miserable month!

The next year there were further tests for us both. Sam had two operations to check if there were any sperm that might then be used in IVF. The second of these operations was carried out alongside a round of IVF drugs for me so that any sperm could be used immediately. Before taking all this on we had read a lot, attempting to work out as best we could whether it would be possible to proceed in a way that respected God. We found John Wyatt's book *Matters of Life and Death* especially helpful. Eventually we decided to aim to fertilise a fairly low number of eggs, with the intention of giving them all a chance to implant at some stage.

Although there is debate about the ethics of freezing embryos as some do not survive, we considered the situation not hugely dissimilar to the fact that month by month many embryos will be fertilised but fail to implant, or miscarry very quickly. So whilst convinced that each one is a unique human life created by God, it was our view that those lost in the freezing process were certainly not being intentionally killed and therefore this remained in line with God's desire for us to honour his right to give and take life. However, we certainly would not claim to have the final answer on this, and can see a lot of wisdom in those we know who have taken different approaches. At one point we felt quite paralysed about the decision, knowing it was good to desire birth children but not wanting to be disobedient to God. A friend, knowing we had prayed and prayed, searched the Bible carefully, examined our motives, and sought godly advice on the issue, reminded us that we could trust God to make our paths straight as we sought to submit to him (eg Proverbs 3:5-6). Not that the final outcome suggests God was not pleased for us to undertake IVF, but we felt secure that he would ensure the right outcome for us and for his glory.

The result of the second operation was negative; no sperm was found. For us that was the end of the line in terms of birth children. Whilst we were aware of Christians who had used donor sperm, we had agreed this was not something we wanted to do, perhaps especially because the idea of adoption was ticking away in the back of our minds, and we felt for us it would be easier to parent with a similar genetic relationship to the child. In this respect we recognise we had an easier time than many infertile couples, as there was a degree of relief in having a clear end to the pursuit of birth children. For others things will be much less clear.

The next couple of months were a time of mourning, getting our heads round the difference between God's plan and ours. We were so thankful to have been clearly taught about God's loving sovereign control in our lives, and the certainty we could have of his love for us through Jesus's life, death and resurrection. I prayed God might take away my desire for birth children and around mid-February I remember noticing my feelings were changing. The loss was less raw, and I found that Psalm 131:1-2 seemed to describe my experience of learning to entrust myself to God and his goodness: 'My heart is not proud, Lord, my eyes are not haughty; I do not concern myself with great matters or things too wonderful for me. But I have calmed and quietened myself, I am like a weaned child with its mother; like a weaned child I am content.' This doesn't mean the pain of infertility disappeared, but there was certainly a change and an acceptance that God had better plans and wanted to do good to us. This made it possible to think clearly about adoption. We found places on introductory days about international and domestic adoption in the spring. We were keen to proceed with domestic adoption, and so applied to social services and in June started the first part of the assessment, followed by about ten visits from a social worker to our home to discuss pretty much every aspect of our lives. Our assessment was completed quite quickly and we were approved as adopters by early December 2010.

Many people have had different experiences from ours in terms of this process. Some people ask whether we felt at a disadvantage as Christians. I actually feel there are many advantages for Christians. As people who know we are saved by grace we were willing to speak about our weaknesses without being defensive and also to be non-judgmental of what we read of the lives of the kind of birth families our children might come from. Equally, church is a wonderful support network which social services are always interested in. Overall, we felt we should be asked careful questions, as the children we might be caring for deserved the process to be thorough.

After approval as adopters, we waited to be 'matched' – chosen as the best option for a particular child. The three or four month wait seemed like years, but eventually we were matched with twin girls who were nine months old. We met the girls in their foster home, and then the ball was in our court as to whether we wanted to proceed. We very much did but also felt it was important to think through our ability to take on the rather intimidating prospect of twins, and there were also some medical uncertainties we needed to have investigated before the match could be approved. The match was finally approved in June 2011. We then had two weeks of 'introductions' which involved lots of visits to the foster home, getting to know the girls and trying to minimise the disruption and confusion they would inevitably experience. They finally moved in a few days before their first birthday.

Since then things have been a bit of a blur! Taking care of twins doesn't provide much time for reflection. There were lots of visits from social workers reviewing how things were going until about October when they were happy for us to apply for the adoption to be finalised by a judge. After this we went for a special day in court where the girls were given new birth certificates and made part of our family forever.

Today, most of life is like any family. The girls bring huge joy to us and many other people. They are great fun and share a close relationship. I can't say what it feels like to love a birth child but I know we love our girls and they love us. We did have to get to know each other (although I guess that happens with birth children too) and as we were committed to loving them, our feelings deepened gradually. They are also very normal in their tantrums, disobedience, and everything else you might expect from a three-year-old. We are thankful they seem well settled and attached to us, as that is not always straightforward for adopted children. We're glad we had time to settle in together as a family over a quiet summer.

I think it is important to grasp that adoption isn't the answer to the pain of infertility. Adoption exists because of loss, primarily the loss experienced by children whose birth parents, for whatever reason, cannot care for them. Often it proceeds from the loss infertile couples experience as they let go of the idea of birth children, although we pray experienced parents might also be willing to meet the needs of children in the care system.

It has been challenging to us to recognise how easily we could want to be parents in order to meet our needs, to ease our pain, rather than for God's glory and the good of our children. The girls do meet our needs, because God made us to flourish when we love others as he loves us. But adoption cuts right to the heart of any selfish attitudes. You have to grasp that these children are not there to fill the hole left by the expectations you may have had of birth children; adoption forces you to face up to this issue.

Adoption is a wonderful opportunity for our own stumbling imitation of God's gracious adoption of us into his family. But there are big differences. Our adoption by God is by a perfect parent, and involves only gain. Human adoption involves flawed parents and children who have experienced a fundamental and significant loss. It's not something we think about all the time, and day by day our girls are very happy little things, but it does surface in various ways. We won't help our girls by trying to make it seem like they are lucky to have ended up in our amazing family.

We hope we can teach them and God can give them faith to trust his loving hand in the messy aspects of their lives. Equally, whilst our own desire for children is certainly met in our girls, the feeling of being different and the pain that sometimes entails is still there, especially in our current stage of life in toddler groups and endless rounds of pregnancies and breast-feeding conversations. I don't feel as intensely bitter or sad as I have previously, but there remains sadness that surfaces at times. I also increasingly grasp some of the pain an adopted child has to come to terms with, and although these issues are less on the surface for Sam, they have not disappeared through adoption. We are learning that God uses this ongoing pain to keep us dependent on him and looking forward to a new creation. Our experience has taught us that God had plans for us we couldn't possibly have imagined and which are a lot more interesting than what we had come up with!

GLOSSARY OF TERMS

Embryo
The living individual that develops from the moment an egg and sperm fuse until eight weeks gestation in the womb.

Egg / Ovum
Female sex cell produced in the ovaries. This does not have the same status as an embryo. It is not a unique human being. In fact before fertilisation with a sperm cell this is more like a skin cell except that it has only half the number of chromosomes.

Fertilisation
Begins with contact between sperm and egg, which then fuse, leading to maturation of the egg and fusion of both nuclei. Process ends with cleavage and formation of the two-cell embryo.

Fetus
Term used for the developing baby in the womb from eight weeks to birth.

Gamete
Term used to denote either egg or sperm cell.

Sperm
Male sex cell produced in the testes. This does not have the same status as an embryo. It is not a unique human being. Before fertilisation with an egg its status is more like a skin cell except that it has only half the number of chromosomes.

FURTHER RESOURCES

BOOKS AND ARTICLES

- Beer D., ed. *Christian choices in healthcare*. Leicester: CMF and IVP, 1995
- Best M. *Fearfully and wonderfully made: ethics and the beginning of human life*. Australia: Matthias Media, 2012.
- Commission on Parenthood's Future. My daddy's name is donor. *bit.ly/yjTuf9*
- McCarthy B. *Fertility and faith: the ethics of human fertilization.* Leicester: Inter-Varsity Press, 1997.
- McWhinnie A., ed. *Who am I? Experiences of donor conception.* Leamington Spa: Idreos Education Trust, 2006.
- Saunders, P. Infertility treatments. *Nucleus*. Spring 2003:13-21. *cmf.li/13G9rHU*
- Wyatt J. *Matters of life and death: Human dilemmas in the light of the Christian faith*. Revised edition, Leicester: CMF and IVP, 2009.

CMF FILES

The *CMF Files* are ethics papers dealing with specific issues. They are available to download from: *www.cmf.org.uk/publications/cmf-files*

- Taylor P. Surrogacy. *CMF File* 47, 2012
- Campbell M. The family and bioethics. *CMF File* 38, 2009
- Berry C. Artificial reproduction. *CMF File* 6, 1999

ADOPTION

- Moore R. *Adopted for Life*. Wheaton, Illinois: Crossway, 2009

- Piper J. Adoption: the heart of the gospel. *bit.ly/atbhhl*

WEBSITES

- Christian Medical Fellowship: *www.cmf.org.uk*

- Life FertilityCare Programme – an alternative to IVF: *www.lifefertilitycare.co.uk*

- Fertility Care Centres of Europe website – for more information on NaPro Technology: *www.fertilitycare.net*

- The Human Fertilisation and Embryology Authority: *www.hfea.gov.uk*

- The National Institute for Health and Care Excellence: *www.nice.org.uk*

REFERENCES

1. In IVF, eggs are removed from the ovaries and fertilised with sperm in a laboratory dish before being placed in the woman's womb. IVF literally means 'fertilisation in glass', giving us the familiar term 'test tube baby'.
2. You may also like to read Jubraj R and Jubraj B. *Infertility - the silent and unseen issue*. Weybridge, Surrey: Roper Penberthy, 2007, who come to a different conclusion about IVF to us (that it is not ethically wise to use it).
3. *Three things are never satisfied; four never say 'enough': Sheol, the barren womb, the land never satisfied with water, and the fire that never says, 'Enough'*. (Proverbs 30:15b-16). The bitterness that Hannah experienced is connected elsewhere in the Bible with the pain of one's own children dying (eg Ruth 1:13, 20; 2 Kings 4:27). Before Rachel eventually bore children she said to Jacob, *'Give me children, or I shall die!'* (Genesis 30:1).
4. The Church of Scotland Board of Social Responsibility. *Pre-conceived ideas: a Christian perspective of IVF and embryology*. Edinburgh: Saint Andrews Press, 1996:14
5. Note that 75% of couples who conceive with this technique do so within 12 months (93% within 18 months) but it may take up to 24 months. For women nearing the end of their reproductive years this may be a disadvantage of this approach. In addition it is not suitable for those whose infertility problem arises from azoospermia (no measurable sperm in the semen), ovarian failure, or bilateral fallopian tube occlusion. See Stanford JB, Parnell TA, Boyle PC. Outcomes from treatment of infertility with natural procreative technology in an Irish general practice. *J Am Board Fam Med* 2008;21:375-384
6. *Ibid*. See also: Tham E, Schliep K, Stanford J. Natural procreative technology for infertility and recurrent miscarriage: outcomes in a Canadian family practice. *Can Fam Physician* 2012;58:267-74. For three case studies see: Boyle P, Stanford J. Naprotechnology (natural procreative technology) - a multifactorial approach to the chronic problem of infertility. *Biomedicina* 2011;21:61-68
7. See, for example: Romans 8:15, 23; Galatians 4:5; Ephesians 1:5
8. 2 Timothy 3:16-17
9. Genesis 16-21
10. 1 Samuel 1
11. Genesis 4:1. '[Eve] said: "*With the help of the Lord I have brought forth a man*"'. In Genesis 16:2 Sarah (or Sarai) acknowledged that it was God who had prevented her having children.
12. Psalm 24:1
13. Psalm 127 and 128
14. Genesis 1:28
15. Saunders P. Infertility treatments. *Nucleus*. Spring 2003:13-21 *cmf.li/13G9rHU*
16. Or had twelve cycles of artificial insemination. Updated NICE guidelines. 2013 *bit.ly/13FN1GM*
17. NICE Guidance. Fertility: assessment and treatment for people with fertility problems. *bit.ly/27Muka*
18. An ultrasound probe is inserted into the vagina to identify follicles. A thin needle is inserted into an ultrasound guide to go through the vagina and into the follicles to retrieve the eggs.
19. Note that 'success' rates vary between clinics. An alternative IVF procedure is intrauterine insemination (IUI). With IUI, before fertility treatment starts, the best quality sperm are selected and are then inserted into the womb at the woman's most fertile time, when an ovary releases an egg (ovulation). This aims to maximise the number of healthy sperm reaching the fallopian tubes and fertilising an egg. IUI often takes place alongside ovarian stimulation to increase egg production and improve the rate of success. In some cases, egg selection may be suggested. This enables only the healthiest eggs to be taken from the ovaries for fertilisation outside the body and can be useful for women with a diminished number and quality of eggs. With gamete intra-fallopian transfer (GIFT), eggs are removed from the ovaries and the healthiest are selected and placed together with sperm in the woman's fallopian tubes. Fertilisation therefore takes place in the body, as it would if fertilisation had occurred naturally. See HFEA. Your fertility treatment options. *bit.ly/192PETX*
20. Over half (52.9% in 2011) of fresh treatments for infertility now involve ICSI. HFEA. Fertility treatment in 2011: trends and figures. *bit.ly/192QcZU*
21 HFEA: *bit.ly/199Z4Ar*
22. Vaughan D et al. Delivery outcomes for nulliparous women at the extremes of maternal age - a cohort study. *BJOG*. June 2013. *bit.ly/14jOLHk*. Also HFEA. Risks of IVF. *bit.ly/14y2sUa*
23. Kennedy R. Risks and complications of assisted conception. 2005 *bit.ly/17x59Ak*. Women who undergo infertility treatment are more likely to develop a serious complication in pregnancy, research suggests: *1.usa.gov/15KDksl*. Some research has also shown a greater risk of ovarian tumours later in life: *1.usa.gov/142Rgl6*
24. HFEA. Embryo transfer and multiple births. *bit.ly/11LSScl*
25. The HFEA states that: 'babies are more likely to be

premature and to have a below-normal birth weight. Studies show that the risk of death before birth, or within the first week of life, is more than four times greater for twins than for a single baby. For triplets, the risk is seven times greater than for a single baby. The risk of cerebral palsy is five times higher for twins and 18 times higher for triplets than for a single baby.' HFEA. Risks of fertility treatment. *bit.ly/14j1KHw* also see *bit.ly/16u645p*

26. HFEA. Fertility treatment in 2011: trends and figures. *bit.ly/192QcZU*
27. HFEA. Fertility drugs. *bit.ly/199WtGM*
28. Ovarian hyperstimulation syndrome. *1.usa.gov/LOAG7N*
29. IVF involves some risk to newly created embryos and is associated with an increased incidence of birth defects according to, for example, one large study that found the risk of a birth defect is 5.8% following natural conception, compared with 7.2% following IVF and 9.9% after ICSI. Davies M *et al*. Reproductive technologies and the risk of birth defects. *New Engl J Med* 2012;366:1803-1813. *bit.ly/JTQpEK*. ICSI was introduced in 1992 so the HFEA states that it is not yet known whether there is any risk that injecting the sperm into an egg could damage it, with possible long-term consequences for the child. However research from Australia has found that one in ten children conceived using the fertility treatment ICSI have birth defects. *bit.ly/16zbDSb* Also Davies M. *et al*. *Op Cit*.
30. HFEA. Fertility treatment risks. *bit.ly/14j1KHw*
31. HFEA. Multiple births and single embryo transfer review. *bit.ly/14j4qEU*. Note that this risk also applies to multiple pregnancies which occur naturally.
32. Braude P. One child at a time: reducing multiple births after IVF. 2006. *bit.ly/15NpOIE*
33. Ord T. The scourge: moral implications of natural embryo loss. *Am J Bioeth* 2008;8:13. *bit.ly/8YnGWR*
34. This does not mean that it is *morally good* to kill embryos. One would not assume that since God allows natural disasters like flooding to occur in Bangladesh that human life is of less value there. It is painful and confusing to ponder that in a fallen world so many human lives are lost so early and yet in his sovereignty the all-knowing God allows this tragedy.
35. Sandel M. Embryo ethics - the moral logic of stem-cell research. *New Engl J Med* 2004;351:208. Sandel argues against the personhood of the embryo but highlights that the comparable risk of IVF to natural embryo loss is often used to defend its practice.
36. Deliberately discarding, rather than implanting embryos, which IVF often involves, is an entirely different matter.
37. If an embryo has stopped dividing in optimum conditions we consider this to be a sign that the embryo has died (we are using the word 'viable' in that sense). Embryos dividing slowly or sub-optimally are still potentially viable and in our view should be treated as weak and vulnerable human beings.
38. If more are produced then the 'best' embryo can be chosen and others could be frozen for further attempts. The logic of this approach is that it avoids having to harvest more eggs and go through the fertilisation process again.
39. The AV and RSV translations of the original Hebrew implied different punishments for the accidental killing of a mother (death penalty) and her unborn child (a fine). The conclusion has sometimes in the past therefore been that God himself apportioned different values to mother and fetus. The NIV translation, by contrast, implies that the death penalty was for fetal or maternal death, and the fine was for injury *without* fetal or maternal death. This latter interpretation is now accepted as the correct one by most contemporary scholars. Even if the former interpretation were correct, the fact is that the text deals with accidental, not deliberate, killing. We cannot therefore infer from this text that the early fetus or embryo is worth less in the eyes of God, or that it can be justifiably killed.
40. Some may object that no parallels can be drawn between our conception and Christ's. Yet we know Jesus was fully human because the Bible tells us that he *'shared in their humanity'* and was *'like us in every way'*, except that he was sinless (Hebrews 2:14-17, 4:15). The significance of this is that the humanity that he took on is our humanity. He had to be one of us in order to be our redeemer. The mode of conception of Jesus was unique but the result, in terms of his fully human nature, was identical to our own.
41. Saunders P. Deadly questions...on the status of the embryo. *Nucleus* Autumn 1998:28-34. *cmf.li/165Ah9a*
42. Iglesias T. In vitro fertilisation: the major issues. *J Med Ethics* 1984;1:36-37. Some argue that because up until what is called the 'primitive streak' stage the embryo can divide into twins it is meaningless to speak of a human person before this point. However in these cases the issue is not *whether there is a person*, but *whether there is more than one person*. This does not seem to justify treating the embryo as if there were no persons there.
43. NICE recommendations from 2013 suggest that women under the age of 39 should only have one embryo transferred in their first cycle of IVF but can consider using

two embryos for subsequent cycles. For women aged 40-42 years, double embryo transfer should be considered. *bit.ly/199YqD2*

44. HFEA. Freezing and storing embryos. *bit.ly/13036bY*
45. eg Professor Peter Braude at Guy's and St Thomas' assisted conception unit explains, *'only around two thirds of embryos will survive the freezing and thawing process, and survival will depend mainly on the quality (cleavage stage and morphology) of the embryos.'* Braude P. and Rowell P. Assisted conception III: problems with assisted conception. *BMJ* 2003; 327: 922. Likewise the US Genetics and IVF Institute say that: *'approximately, 65 70% of embryos survive thaw, 10% partially survive and 20-25% are atretic [completely dysfunctional]. Our data suggests that embryos with 100% cell survival are almost as good as embryos never frozen but only about 30-35% survive in this fashion.'* See Genetics and IVF Institute. Human embryo cryopreservation (embryo freezing) and frozen embryo transfer cycles. *bit.ly/cyXgro*
46. The added complication for freezing embryos is that it is impossible to know for certain whether it will be physically possible to implant the embryos into the womb in future for health reasons or whether financial or relational circumstances would make it difficult.
47. The HFEA say that *'to date around 900 babies have been born using frozen eggs worldwide. Only five babies have been born in the UK using frozen eggs...Eggs are known not to respond well to freezing...However, vitrification (a new method for egg storage) has recently been shown to improve the chance of eggs surviving the freeze-thaw process and therefore increase the success rate.'* See HFEA. Freezing and storing embryos. *bit.ly/13036bY*
48. IVF normally involves masturbation at the IVF clinic in order to generate the sperm required for IVF. However some units will give out specific condoms so that people can collect (and if necessary freeze) semen, thereby avoiding masturbation.
49. Frame J. *The doctrine of the Christian life*. Phillipsburg, New Jersey: Presbyterian and Reformed, 2008:767
50. This is developed in more depth in Campbell M. The family and bioethics. *CMF File* 38. 2009
51. Leviticus 18:6-20, 20:10-21
52. Although the donated gamete (the genetic material) will normally be provided anonymously, the child can obtain some information about the identity of their biological father or mother when they are 18. Therefore the longer term social effects of this 'intrusion' cannot be completely ignored.
53. Brendan McCarthy writes *'a couple accept that they are unable to ... experience both the unitive [expression of love] and procreative aspects of sex ... in their marriage ... [so] a woman accepts from another man the means of fulfilment of one aspect of her sexual life without any unitive relationship with him [or vice versa]. The happiness of the woman, and even of her husband should not be minimized, but the price to pay is too great for the practice to be accepted.'* McCarthy B. *Fertility and faith: the ethics of human fertilization*. Leicester: IVP, 1997:183
54. Stott J. The abortion dilemma. *bit.ly/1430gga*
55. Despite the removal of donor anonymity in this country in 2005, donor-conceived people can only find out about their origins if their social parents tell them and many parents choose not to do so. Research suggests that only 10-20% of people who have a child by donor conception have either told that child, or stated that they will at some point tell that child, how he or she was conceived.
56. Genesis 16:1-6, 30:3
57. Taylor P. Surrogacy. *CMF File* 47. 2012
58. In the Bible, the wisdom developed by pagans is sometimes adopted by God's people, eg Acts 7:22. Solomon suggests that the wisdom gained from non-Christian Egyptians can be useful for the God-centred life, eg Proverbs 22:17.
59. HFEA. IVF - chance of success. *bit.ly/199Z4Ar*
60. See *www.lifefertilitycare.co.uk* or *www.fertilitycare.net* for more information on NaPro Technology, an alternative to IVF for couples with infertility.
61. At the time of writing this was still experimental but tremendous progress is being made.
62. To a maximum of two embryos.
63. Sometimes technicians may make wrong assumptions about what you are thinking even when you have discussed details with doctors, eg about how many embryos you would like to be created.
64. Megan Best has a useful section in her book on the advice and support that others can offer to an infertile couple. For example, being there for them (cf Job's friends), keeping comments simple (not trying to fix the problem), being sensitive, not judging or advising, praying, and kind acts, etc. Best also warns about what is less helpful to say and she suggests how to handle comments if on the receiving end. Best M. *Fearfully and wonderfully made: ethics and the beginning of human life*. Kingsford, NSW: Matthias Media. 2012.